I0838088

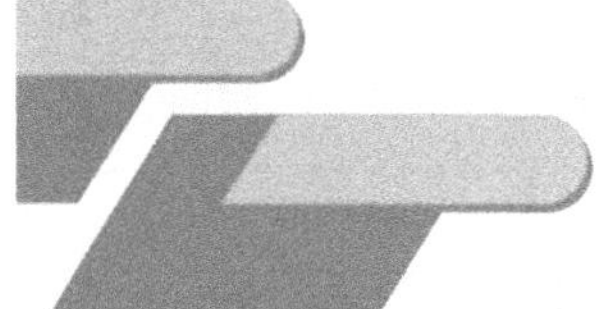

PROVEN EFFECTIVE NATURAL WAYS

TO TREAT ECZEMA

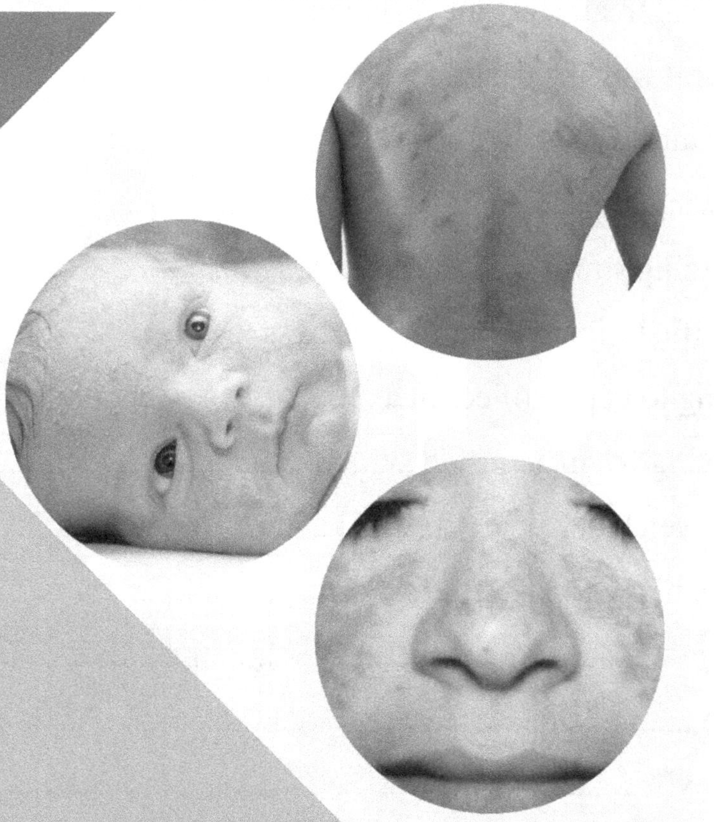

BY MOSES ADROD

TABLE OF CONTENTS

INTRODUCTION

According to the Merriam-Webster online dictionary, eczema is defined as 'an inflammatory condition of the skin characterized by redness, itching and oozing vesicular lesions which become scaly, crusted or hardened'.

This basic dictionary definition immediately gives you some idea that eczema is not a pleasant condition to suffer from.

As we will see as we progress through this book, eczema has been around for thousands of years, but modern medical science is no closer to curing it than our forefathers were.

Like many skin complaints, eczema is one of those things that most people end up treating on a superficial or skin level, primarily because medical science tends to adopt the same attitude.

However, because we are looking for a completely natural way to deal with eczema, many of the solutions you will read about in this book take a much more holistic approach to getting rid of or at least minimizing the worst effects of eczema.

While there are many things you can do on the surface to reduce the severity of eczema using only natural substances, I'm also going to delve into some other ways that you can deal with your eczema from the inside, rather than just the outside.

Before moving on to start looking at various treatments that you can use to deal with your eczema problem, let us look in a little more detail at what the condition is, and who gets it.

WHAT IS ECZEMA?

Like many other skin conditions such as psoriasis and dandruff, there is a great deal about eczema that is still a mystery to us.

For example, because eczema refers to a set of clinical characteristics rather than a single condition, the definition of the underlying causes of eczema has frequently been haphazard and unsystematic (at best). Indeed, many different terms and names have been used for the condition over the years, as dozens of so-called experts have developed their own definitions of what eczema is and is not.

Eczema is frequently confused with psoriasis, which is due in part to this confusion. The two conditions are not identical, with the main difference being that adult eczema is frequently found on the flexor aspect of body joints (those body parts on the inside of a joint that can decrease in size or surface area due to flexing), whereas psoriasis is not.

What is generally agreed is that eczema is a form of dermatitis. Dermatitis in turn is used as a 'catch-all' term for any inflammation of the epidermis, which is the outermost layer of the human skin.

Consequently, for many non-medical professionals, the two words eczema and dermatitis are almost interchangeable, and (just to confuse things a little further) you will also hear eczema referred to as eczematous dermatitis or dermatitis eczema.

Eczema is frequently confused with psoriasis, which is due in part to this confusion. The two conditions are not identical, with the main difference being that adult eczema is frequently found on the flexor aspect of body joints (those body parts on the inside of a joint that can decrease in size or surface area due to flexing), whereas psoriasis is not.

WHO CAN SUFFER FROM ECZEMA?

The answer to the question is, anyone can suffer from eczema.

While it most commonly begins in a baby or child, it can affect men and women, young and old, and is not limited to those in their first few years of life.

Although each person's symptoms vary, eczema is typically characterized by dry, red patches of skin that are extremely itchy. Unfortunately, because the natural tendency is to scratch any itch, no matter how much you know you shouldn't, eczema is sometimes referred to as 'itch that can cause rashes' because scratching an itch results in a rash more often than not.

Eczema usually appears as dry red patches on the cheeks, forehead, scalp, neck, forearms, and legs in babies and children. Fortunately, most children's eczema gradually fades as they grow, so many children who had eczema as babies or toddlers will have no problems as adults.

Many factors, however, can trigger an outbreak of eczema in adults who have been free of the condition for many years. In adults, the dry red skin is most commonly found on the insides of the elbows, knees, and, less frequently, the ankles. Simultaneously, the condition can flare up and exhibit many of the symptoms associated with childhood eczema.

Being a chronic condition, there is no known cure for eczema although the condition is generally not dangerous. In addition, there are plenty of different ways of treating it.

However, because children find it difficult not to scratch, it is not uncommon for children with eczema to break the skin, making them far more susceptible to infections and other conditions that attack broken skin, such as warts.

TYPES OF ECZEMA

There are several types of eczema, each of which is thought to have a unique cause. As a result, the cause of eczema is determined by the type of condition that the sufferer has.

The main types of eczema that you are likely to come across are as follows, with the most widely accepted causes of each different type listed in the description.

Atopic eczema: The most common type of eczema is atopic eczema, which is thought to be a hereditary condition. The condition is sometimes referred to as infantile eczema because, due to its hereditary nature, it is most commonly seen in children.

If one parent has eczema, or if they have hay fever (the strongest indicator) or asthma, the child has a much higher chance of having eczema. In fact, if both parents have eczema, their child's chances of developing the condition are as high as 80%.

If your child has atopic eczema, it is thought that their immune system is overreacting to some kind of external stimulus, such as pollen, dust mites, animal hair, or skin flakes, resulting in irritated, inflamed, and (most importantly) itchy skin.

If a child is suffering from atopic eczema, they will exhibit most of the classical eczema conditions mentioned earlier, such as itchy red lesions on the head, neck, scalp and face and the flexor areas of the body.

If these skin lesions are scratched with sufficient severity, it is likely that the skin will bleed, raising the possibility of suffering infections.

Another issue is that many people with eczema scratch their skin until it becomes tough, leathery, and hard. These lesions can occasionally dry out, resulting in the dry, flaky skin that eczema patients are accustomed to.

Fortunately, none of these particular aspects of suffering atopic eczema represent any kind of serious medical problem, although if the skin is broken and infections enter the body, the story might be very different.

However, as any eczema sufferer will tell you, the itching that is perhaps the best-known 'symptom' of the condition can drive you crazy.

Although of course adult eczema sufferers know better than to keep scratching the patches of eczema, this does not mean that they can resist the urge when the itching becomes extreme.

The situation is far worse for children. It is much more difficult to persuade a child to stop scratching, especially since recent research suggests that there is a scientific basis for believing that scratching an itch actually provides relief.

Another 'symptom' of atopic eczema seen in some patients is a tendency for children's ears to discharge a mixture of mucus, ear wax, or even blood. This is most common in children who have dry eczema on the surface of or just inside their ears.

This is nothing to be particularly concerned about, nor is it unusual, but if blood is present in the discharge, it may be prudent to seek medical advice so that you can at least establish the cause of the problem.

Finally, as previously stated, there is strong evidence that atopic eczema is exacerbated by a weakened immune system. As a result, it makes sense to do everything possible to strengthen your immune system in order to fight the condition.

Contact dermatitis: This is a form of eczema that is caused by contact with irritants that can trigger an eczema flare-up.

The reactions that you might suffer as a contact dermatitis sufferer can be categorized in one of two ways.

In the first example, irritant contact dermatitis is a condition that comes on extremely quickly after you have been exposed to a chemical substance that immediately irritates the skin.

Irritant contact dermatitis accounts for approximately 75% of all cases of contact dermatitis. This is because the condition is one of the most common industrial diseases experienced by employees in many industrialized Western countries. It should come as no surprise that those who work in heavy industry, such as chemical manufacturing or iron smelting, frequently suffer from contact dermatitis, even if the individual employee has no prior history or family history of similar problems.

The second type of contact dermatitis is known as allergen contact dermatitis, meaning that the individual concerned suffers a delayed reaction to previous contact with an allergen like poison ivy, pollen etc

These two types of contact dermatitis do not have to be mutually exclusive. It is possible to have both types of contact dermatitis and possibly atopic eczema at the same time, depending on the strength of an individual's immune system.

Xerotic eczema: This is a rare form of eczema caused by dry skin (often seasonal) that has become so dry and cracked that eczema lesions begin to form. This condition is more common in older people, with the limbs and torso being the most commonly affected areas.

Less common forms of eczema: In addition to the three most common types of eczema listed above, there are many other less widely known and less common variations of the condition.

These are as follows:

Dyshidrosis: This condition only affects the palms, soles of your feet, and the sides of your fingers. This type of eczema is distinguished by tiny bumps known as vesicules and skin cracks that itch more during the night than during the day.

Although it is not common in comparison to atopic or contact eczema, Dyshidrosis is probably the most common hand eczema, one which worsens when the weather gets warmer.

Discoid eczema: In contrast to Dyshidrosis, Discoid eczema is a condition that gets worse in the winter, identified by round red lesions, usually on the lower leg, which can either be excessively dry or oozing.

Neurodermatitis: This is a condition characterized by itchy pigmented, thickened eczema lesions caused most commonly by rubbing and scratching. The treatment for this type of eczema is simple: stop scratching, and the condition will usually go away on its own!

Venous eczema: Venous eczema usually occurs in people who have impaired circulation. It is a condition often seen in people who are over 50 years old, often appearing as a dark, scaly patch of intensely itchy skin in the ankle area. While this type of eczema is not particularly dangerous in and of itself, it can occasionally develop into painful and extremely unpleasant leg ulcers, so if you are in the right age group and notice dark, itchy patches of skin around your ankles, you should seek medical attention.

CAUSES OF ECZEMA

A suggested earlier, it is generally believed that one of the major causes of eczema is a hereditary predisposition to suffering from the condition.

However, there must be some kind of trigger that causes the itchy red skin lesions that are characteristic of eczema to flare up. A flare-up of contact dermatitis, for example, could be triggered by something as seemingly innocuous as wearing rough clothes made of wool or other similarly rough fabrics.

In addition, tobacco smoke, bleach, harsh soaps, pet hair and chemical cosmetics can all trigger an eczema flare up, especially in youngsters who are susceptible to the condition.

Nevertheless, the main cause of most common forms of eczema are hereditary factors, one or both parents having been sufferers from allergic reactions such as asthma - a susceptibility that is somehow passed on to their children.

One strong indicator of this is that in the United States, it is generally agreed that approximately 15% of people (including infants and young children) may suffer from eczema. However, for approximately half of the children included in these statistics, their condition will gradually improve as they grow older, so that by adulthood, they will be free of eczema. In this case, most of the children will grow out of their condition between the ages of 5 and 15 years.

Not everyone is fortunate enough to be completely free of eczema. Adults in the United States with persistent eczema are estimated to account for 5.5% of the adult population, or approximately 15 million US citizens. This means that only one in every three or four children will suffer from childhood eczema into adulthood.

However, the news is not so encouraging everywhere, as a recent report in one of the UK's main quality broadsheets, the Daily Telegraph, reported that cases of eczema had risen by 42% in the four years prior to 2005 in the UK.

The same study published in the Journal of the Royal Society of Medicine suggested that as many as 1 in 9 citizens of the UK had suffered eczema at least once in their life.

The study suggested that one reason could be the modern obsession with soaps and detergents to keep us clean, though it is also likely that another reason could be increased awareness of the condition among both medical professionals and patients themselves, which means that more cases of eczema are being brought to medical attention and classified as eczema than previously.

Other causes

Because so little is known about eczema, there is also a lack of detailed scientific knowledge about other factors that can cause an eczema flare-up. What causes a major flare-up of the condition in one person will leave another completely untouched, as you will read on many eczema websites. As a result, it is extremely difficult to predict what will cause an eczema attack in any particular person.

However, there are many factors which are believed to exacerbate the condition in those who are regular sufferers. There are therefore life changes that you can make that should reduce your tendency to suffer flare-ups of eczema.

Let's consider the most widely stated causes of eczema as a way of starting to investigate how you can deal with your eczema problem completely naturally.

Your diet

While many medical professionals will treat a patient's eczema problem on a topical basis, from a 'natural treatment' standpoint, it is often better to treat the condition on a 'holistic' whole body basis, as suggested in the introduction to this book. To put it another way, treating a medical condition or problem from the inside out is always more effective than the other way around, and eczema is no exception.

There are many foodstuffs that are believed to exacerbate eczema. It is therefore logical to consider changing your diet to remove any of the foodstuffs that are believed to bring on eczema or to make the condition worse.

Before doing so, it is important to understand that eczema is a condition that affects everyone differently. There is no way to know for certain which of these foods will have a negative impact on you because everyone reacts differently to their own diet.

As the saying puts it, 'one man's meat is another man's poison'. Consequently, there is no way that you can remove any particular type of food from your diet with 100% certainty that doing so will help to alleviate your eczema problem.

Nevertheless, it is generally believed that many of the foods in the following list can make your eczema considerably worse. What you therefore need to do is experiment, and try removing certain foods from your diet or from the diet of your children if it is they that suffer from eczema.

However, you should gradually eliminate certain foods from your diet or that of your family, because if you try to change everything at once and see a significant improvement, you will have no idea which foods were previously causing the problem.

While it might be a little frustrating having to be patient while changing your diet, to gain any meaningful results from your 'diet change experiment', you have to change one thing at a time.

This is often referred to as following an elimination diet, in which you remove one specific group of foods from your diet and avoid that food group for at least two or three weeks. You should keep a detailed diary during this time to record what is happening in terms of eczema flare-ups and other potential problems.

The basic idea is that if your eczema problem improves by a significant margin while you are avoiding certain foodstuffs only to return when you start reintroducing them to your diet, you have isolated a dietary problem that is exacerbating your eczema.

These are the food groups to work on:

Wheat based products: Wheat flour, which is typically high in gluten, is used in foods such as bread, biscuits, and pretzels. Gluten, like the other foods on this list, is thought to trigger eczema flare-ups, so try eliminating gluten-based products from your diet for a while. Coffee substitutes, beer, and root beer may all contain grain as well as yeast, which is also a component of most bread products.

Yeast is a fungus, one that has sometimes been indicated to be a potential cause of eczema. Try removing yeast-based products from your diet to see what difference (if any) doing so makes.

Dairy products: The dairy product family, which includes milk (from cows, goats, or sheep), as well as milk-containing foods like yoghurt, cheese, and ice cream, is perhaps the most commonly associated with causing eczema. It is even suggested that processed milk-containing foods, such as chocolate, pastries, and soups, be avoided because it is widely accepted that dairy products are frequently one of the major causes of eczema.

It is believed that babies who are naturally breast-fed are far less likely to suffer from eczema than is a baby who takes formula milk.

If Mum intends to breast-feed, she should limit her intake of dairy products during pregnancy. This is because trace elements of the substances that are present in milk which apparently cause outbreaks of eczema (such as whey protein, lactose sugar and casein protein) will be passed from mother to baby if she consumes too many dairy products while pregnant.

Fish and seafood: Oily fish like salmon, tuna, trout, mackerel and sardines have all been implicated in causing eczema flare-ups. While oily fish is generally extremely good for you because it contains the essential omega-3 fatty acids (which have been shown to help to combat depression, cancer and heart disease), these fatty acids can sometimes cause problems for eczema sufferers.

However, there are no hard and fast rules about what particular foods will cause an eczema-sufferer problem and which will help them. This is especially true of omega-3 fatty acids, which can often help reduce inflammation in all areas of the body rather than causing it. Because eczema is a skin inflammation condition, it is possible that some people will benefit rather than suffer from including omega-3 in their diet.

Given the degree of uncertainty, if you want to try including fish oil in your diet to increase the levels of omega-3, you must keep a very close record of your results (remember the elimination diet notion).

I would also recommend that you use supplements rather than trying to eat lots of oily fish. This is because many predator oily fish (those that get the omega-3 from eating other fish, like salmon, mackerel and albacore tuna) also tend to eat lots of toxins at the same time.

As an example, it is increasingly common for salmon and tuna to be very high in mercury and dioxins, so if you want to include larger amounts of omega-3 in your diet, use provably safe supplements to do so.

Crustaceans such as lobster, crab, prawns, and crayfish, as well as mollusks (clams, oysters, mussels, and so on), are also thought to be foods to avoid. While the jury is still out on whether eating oily fish is good for people with eczema, there is little doubt that shellfish and crustaceans are almost always a problem for people with eczema.

Acidic fruits: Research has indicated that including acidic fruits such as cranberries, blueberries and currants will cause an increased level of eczema affected skin production in many sufferers.

Canned or glazed fruits will often cause problems as well, primarily because in the canning or glazing process, artificial preservatives are very commonly used.

Nuts: All 'true' nuts like almonds, pistachios, cushion nuts, hazelnuts and walnuts have the ability to make eczema far worse if they are included in your diet. Peanuts are often believed to cause problems for anyone who has eczema, despite the fact that a peanut is not in fact a nut at all (it's a legume, similar to beans and peas).

If you are particularly sensitive to peanuts as a cause of eczema, it is critical that you check processed or pre-packaged foods for peanut traces. While the practice of including peanut extract or traces in processed or pre-packaged foods has decreased significantly in recent years, you should still check to ensure that anything you eat does not contain peanut residue if peanuts are a major concern.

Eggs: Eggs and other foodstuffs that are either based on or use eggs in the creation or manufacturing process should be avoided as well. As an example, cakes often contain eggs, so cakes should be avoided.

Egg allergies are common, with some sources suggesting that an allergy to eggs and egg materials is one of the most common causes of atopic eczema in children.

Don't forget the idea of the elimination diet. If you suspect that eggs are causing a problem, eliminate them from your diet for a while before gradually reintroducing them. If your eczema symptoms reappear, you will have a much clearer picture of what is causing you problems.

Food additives, colorings and preservatives: Many of the better-known and more commonly used food additives, colorings and preservatives can also cause your eczema to flare-up.

The majority of foods we eat and beverages we drink contain preservatives or additives of some kind, but you should try to avoid consuming foods or drinks that are high in chemical additives as much as possible.

As an example, substances like tartrazine, monosodium glutamate and sodium benzoate are all known to be capable of irritating your system to the extent that you suffer a flare-up of eczema.

These chemical-based food additives can never be considered natural. As a result, if you want to get rid of your eczema completely naturally, you should avoid foods that contain these preservatives or colorings.

ALLERGY TESTING TO ESTABLISH WHAT CAUSES ECZEMA

As previously stated, one of the most common causes of eczema is an allergic reaction or the fact that a particular person is especially susceptible to specific allergens such as tree pollen, pet hair, and so on.

Furthermore, we established in the previous chapter that many eczema sufferers are prone to allergic reactions to certain foodstuffs which can prompt a flare-up of the condition at any time.

I have mentioned that one way of discovering what particular foodstuffs or beverages cause you eczema problems is to keep a journal of your elimination diet.

Doing things this way has the advantage that you can do everything in the comfort of your own home and there is no need to spend money for anything other than the diary that you use.

Another option for determining what is causing your eczema flare-ups is to undergo an allergy test under medical supervision. This test should reveal exactly what you are allergic to, though it may take some time to see positive results because the allergist you are working with may have identified many different allergens to which you may be reacting, implying that their testing may be slow.

On the other hand, taking an allergy test is not only effective for highlighting those foodstuffs or chemicals in food that you react against. It will also highlight any non-dietary factors that might be causing your eczema, such as an allergy to dust mites, tobacco smoke or even to the chemicals in strong soap and detergents.

In short, allergy testing is a far more comprehensive way of determining exactly what is causing your eczema problem, because an allergy test will also establish an individual's personal reactions to various allergens such as tree pollen, molds, or medications, in addition to allergies.

On the other hand, because allergy testing only establishes that the tested individual has a specific allergic antibody to the particular substance being tested, it does not necessarily mean that an allergic reaction is the inevitable result of the presence of these antibodies.

For example, while an allergy test may reveal that a specific individual has antibodies that are likely to react to substances such as pet hair or dust mites, this does not necessarily imply that they will be allergic or react to these specific allergens.

Consequently, if you are going to use allergy testing to establish what causes your eczema problem, you need to have a test that can be analyzed and interpreted by a qualified board certified allergist (in the USA – qualified UK allergists are listed here).

When you first begin working with an allergist, they will most likely ask you a lot of questions about your lifestyle in order to determine the most likely causes of your adverse reactions to allergens, foods that you are allergic to, and so on. For example, they will inquire about your family history, because, as previously stated, problems such as eczema are thought to have a hereditary component.

In general, there are only two types of allergy testing that are commonly accepted as being scientifically valid for anything other than experimental research purposes.

The first is the skin test, which has been used for over a century and is still the preferred method of allergy testing today. In this case, the qualified practitioner applies a small drop of a commercially prepared solution containing the allergen to which the patient is suspected of being allergic to the skin before scratching the skin, allowing the allergen to enter the body.

When doing so, the allergist will be looking for a specific degree or level of reaction from the patient to demonstrate that they are sensitive to a specific allergen. However, because the initial allergen solution is so weak, it is common for the allergist to perform several skin tests with slightly stronger allergen solutions to determine the severity of the patient's adverse reaction.

The allergist is artificially inducing an allergic disease in miniature. If the initial test on the outside of the skin is not effective for establishing exactly what it is that is causing some kind of negative reaction, a similar test will be run by injecting the allergen solution under the skin.

The alternative form of allergy testing is known as Radioallergosorbent testing (RAST), which is a test for specific allergic antibodies in the blood, a test which is gradually improving in scope and accuracy.

However, because RAST is considerably more expensive than skin testing and because the results often take days or even weeks to arrive, it is still skin testing that is by far the most popular form of allergy test.

With an allergy test, you may be able to get a much clearer picture of why you have eczema or other complaints that are more common in those who appear to be more prone to allergic reactions. With this information, it is much easier to determine the changes you need to make in your life to reduce your susceptibility (or that of your children) to eczema.

MEDICAL TREATMENTS FOR ECZEMA

The appearance of a patient's skin, as well as their family and personal history, are commonly used to make a clinical diagnosis of eczema.

However, because there are many conditions that are similar to eczema (for example, psoriasis), your doctor will need to examine your skin lesions to rule out other issues.

They may even need to perform a skin lesion biopsy to determine exactly what you are suffering from, though this is unlikely in most cases.

Once your medical practitioner has determined that you do indeed have eczema, they will most likely recommend a variety of treatment options based on the severity of your eczema problem.

Nevertheless, irrespective of what kind of treatment they prescribe for you, the ultimate objectives of the treatment will always be the same:

- To control and reduce itching;
- To reduce skin inflammation;
- To loosen and then remove scaly skin lesions;
- To reduce the outbreak of new lesions; and
- To clear any infection that has already set in.

There are many strategies that your doctor may recommend you use to reduce the severity of your problem, such as moisturizing your skin (more on that later), applying topical pharmaceuticals, or, in more severe cases, taking oral medications.

Most commonly, the medications that will be prescribed for treating your eczema are likely to be based on corticosteroids, a type of steroid hormone that is naturally produced in the adrenal cortex.

Most doctors will recommend a corticosteroid-based topical cream or ointment as a first-line treatment for eczema as a first option. Many such corticosteroid creams are available without a prescription in Western countries, implying (quite correctly) that the creams you purchase are not particularly potent.

They are unlikely to have any particularly adverse side-effects either, but their effectiveness may be fairly limited.

If your condition continues to deteriorate or does not improve, your doctor may prescribe you a corticosteroid cream or lotion, meaning that this particular topical treatment is likely to be considerably stronger than those that you buy across the counter.

It is widely accepted within the medical community that long-term usage of corticosteroids can have adverse side-effects, such as irreversible skin thinning. Consequently, if your doctor prescribes topical corticosteroid-based lotions or creams, it is likely that they will recommend that you only use them for a short period of time.

The third corticosteroid-based option is for your medical practitioner to recommend oral corticosteroid drugs such as prednisone or prednisolone. While the potential adverse side effects of these drugs will vary depending on the strength of the drug and the length of time you have to take it, there are widely recognized adverse side effects of long-term use of drugs like these.

For example, scroll down the prednisolone page highlighted above and you will see that listed amongst the potential side-effects are weight gain, high blood pressure, worsening of diabetes, glaucoma, diabetes, growth retardation in children and psychic disturbances.

While it is fair to say that it would only be in the most serious of circumstances that a medical practitioner would prescribe a long-term use of corticosteroid drugs like these, it is not impossible that some doctors might do so. Hence, you need to be aware of the dangers of corticosteroid drugs, and if at all possible, avoid using them.

Other pharmaceuticals that might be prescribed by your doctor would be antibiotics in a situation where by scratching the eczema affected areas of your skin you have caused an infection.

When you suffer severe itching as a result of your eczema, you might want to use antihistamines to reduce the severity, with antihistamine-based products being available both across the counter and by prescription.

If you do decide to use antihistamines, keep in mind that one of the side effects of this type of medication is drowsiness. As a result, it is best to take them before going to bed to ensure a good night's sleep. Never be tempted to take them if your job requires you to drive or operate machinery.

Finally, a few years ago, the FDA approved two new drugs that belong to the class known as calcineurin inhibitors, drugs that suppress the activity of your immune system as a way of reducing the worst effects of conditions like eczema.

The two best known 'types' of drugs of this nature are Pimecrolimus (Elidel) and Tacrolimus (Protopic), but because these drugs are still new, there is not as yet a great deal of scientific evidence about any adverse side-effects.

It has been suggested that avoidance of using them helps the kidneys of renal transplant patients to function far more efficiently, which would point to the likelihood that there are possible side-effects.

Claims that applying these drugs to the skin can also cause burning and discomfort for several days, with less common side-effects being listed as acne, headaches and possible flu-like symptoms, are a little worrying.

Indeed, the same article claims that the FDA has issued a warning about possible links between topically applied calcineurin inhibitors and cancer. There appears to be little doubt that, like so many others before them, the potential long-term adverse effects of these pharmaceuticals mean that they are not the much-heralded 'wonder drug' that they may have appeared to be at first.

From this chapter, one thing should have become abundantly clear. While your medical practitioner might be able to recommend many chemical-based pharmaceutical treatments for eczema, you would not necessarily want to use any of these particular methods of treatment given the potential adverse side-effects that are inherent in using chemical-based pharmaceuticals.

Because the majority of eczema sufferers have an intermittent problem that is not particularly serious aside from the highly irritating itching, even medical practitioners are frequently happy to recommend natural solutions that you can try before resorting to pharmaceuticals.

Let us consider some of these natural options next.

NATURAL WAYS OF DEALING WITH ECZEMA

Moisture is the key

If you are an eczema sufferer who does not have a particularly serious condition, it is possible that you can minimize the effects of eczema to an acceptable level with some practical home-based 'treatments'.

For example, once you've determined what causes your flare-ups (e.g., pollen exposure or food allergies), the solution is to avoid putting yourself in danger. If you know that eggs, milk, or nuts are causing your problem, all you have to do is avoid eating them or try to stay inside during the peak of spring and summer pollen counts.

Given that eczema is a condition that is characterized by dry skin, it is logical that anything that reduces your dry skin is an effective way of dealing with your problem.

For this reason, you should always bathe for as short a time as possible, while also reducing the amount of soap that you use during the bathing process. It will probably be more effective to use a natural moisturizing oil like tea tree oil in your bath because this will help to keep your skin moist and supple.

When you get out of the bath, it is critical that you try to retain as much moisture in your skin as possible by applying natural moisturizers such as olive or tea tree oil to all of your skin's dry areas. Attempt to do this within three minutes of exiting your bath, as doing so ensures that you are applying moisturizer to skin that is still moist and thus flexible.

You can further increase the benefits of this particular strategy by wrapping any dry skin areas to which you have applied moisturizer with plastic bags that will prevent your skin drying out for the maximum length of time.

The primary advantages of using either olive or tea tree oil as a moisturizer is that both of these substances are easy to get hold of.

As with all aspects of dealing with eczema, while these particular moisturizers are highly effective for most people, they may not work for you. Consequently, you might like to consider some alternative moisturizers made from completely natural substances:

Vitamin E oil: Vitamin E oil is well-known for its ability to hydrate the skin while also promoting healing. This moisturizing oil promotes the body's ability to use vitamin K and selenium while also protecting cell membranes. It also adds another layer of protection to your skin due to its antioxidant properties.

Vinca Minor: Vinca minor is a homoeopathic moisturizing solution that is highly effective for relieving sensitive, sore or itchy skin. It is therefore ideal for anyone who suffers from eczema to use as a moisturizer, because dry and itchy skin is probably the most common characteristic of the eczema sufferer.

Hydrocotyle Asiatica: Hydrocotyle is a type of aquatic plant that includes between 75 and 100 different species. However, as a herbal remedy, it has been used for centuries due to its wound healing properties and ability to aid skin rejuvenation. If you can't find moisturizing solutions containing this herb, try looking for it online and infusing it into a mild unscented baby oil to make your own moisturizing solution.

Calendula: Calendula is an ancient medicinal herb which helps to treat dry and damaged skin which is also excellent for minimizing the effects of eczema and psoriasis. In suspension and used topically, calendula is highly effective for reducing skin inflammation while also soothing irritated tissue.

If you search for calendula, you'll find a plethora of stores where you can buy the plants or at least the extract to make your own soothing, moisturizing lotion or oil. In the absence of this, you could consider purchasing a commercially produced calendula salve.

The bottom line is that the more frequently or regularly you can moisturize the affected areas of your skin, the less of a problem you are likely to have. As a result, whenever you wash away layers of moisture from your skin by bathing or showering, you must replace that moisture each time.

Blowing hot and cold:

Extremes of heat or cold are another potential cause of eczema that you should try to avoid whenever possible. While your ability to do so will vary depending on where you live, it is a fact that many people find that extremes of temperature promote eczema flare-ups.

By avoiding temperature extremes, you therefore remove another potential cause of a breakout of eczema.

Avoiding stress: Just take it easy…

People who suffer from stress and tension are more likely to aggravate any pre-existing chronic medical conditions they have, such as eczema and psoriasis, because they allow their emotions to run wild.

If you can reduce stress levels in your life, you will give yourself a far better chance of avoiding further outbreaks of eczema.

The first thing you can do to reduce the amount of stress you have to put up with on a daily basis is to change your life so that you don't put yourself in situations where you are going to be stressed.

For example, if you are the type of person who has to rush to the subway or railway station every morning in order to catch the very last train that will get you to work on time, try getting out of bed 10 minutes earlier so that you can catch a subway or train that is not as desperate.

If you are always too rushed to eat properly because you spend your break times at work, try to get away for 30 minutes or an hour to get away from the stressful environment of work. Even better if you can find a peaceful and relaxing place to visit during your break. Sitting in the park and feeding the ducks is less stressful than fighting your way to the front of the line at your favorite burger or fried food joint.

Try to plan your meals at home in advance as well. By doing so, you ensure that you do not spend every evening immediately after leaving the office having to dash to the mall or convenience store to find food for the family dinner.

If you are constantly at the beck and call of your family, try to make time for yourself to relax and perhaps even pamper yourself. While it is admirable that you will do everything possible to help others, you must recognize that living your life at Mach 3 will harm your health.

When that happens, how will you be able to help and look after others when you are sick?

Stress always floods your body with 'flight or fight' chemicals, which is extremely useful in genuine emergency situations. However, once it becomes a constant factor of your life, it gradually wears you down and further damages your immune system (which as an eczema sufferer is probably in a pretty poor shape anyway) as it does so.

On the other hand, it is unavoidable that if you slow down your daily routine, you will reduce the amount of stress you have to deal with on a daily basis. When you do this, problems that are exacerbated by stress, such as eczema, are likely to become much less problematic for you.

What we are talking about here is a complete reassessment of your life.

You must give yourself the time to take a step back so that you are able to assess everything you do in your normal day-to-day life, because it is only by knowing what you're doing that you can begin to change it.

A daily journal would be invaluable so that you can really see what you do every day. Armed with this information, you can start making the necessary changes to reduce stress levels in your life.

Specific training to minimize stress

In addition to changing your daily routine to reduce the amount of stress that is undoubtedly exacerbating your eczema, there are several things you can learn that may help you to de-stress even more.

In order to learn practices like yoga, it was not all that long ago that you had to go to organized classes which would have cost money, but it is now possible to pick up most of the information that you need from the internet completely free.

This is well worth doing, because practices like yoga have a long history of being used for relaxation as well as for exercise and building strength.

To find as much information as you need about how to start learning to relax properly using yoga, all you need to do is search a major engine like Google using a term like 'learning yoga' or you could look for information about 'yoga for relaxation'. There really is no shortage of yoga information available online, so you can learn everything you need to know in the comfort of your own home.

Combine yoga with other widely accepted practices for slowing down your life and reducing stress, such as learning meditation and proper breathing techniques. By doing so, you can create your own daily relaxation routine that you can use to calm yourself down whenever your stress levels rise.

Remember that this is not about becoming a fully fledged yogi or acknowledge expert in meditation, unless of course you want to. The main focus of what you are doing is to learn new ideas and techniques to ensure that you are always as calm and relaxed as possible.

It is not therefore absolutely necessary to adopt any particular practice in order to achieve a relaxed state, as long as what you find works for you.

For example, the relaxation program outlined on this website combines many different ideas, such as yoga, meditation, and deep breathing, but it is not focused on blind adherence to any particular relaxation regime or stress management ideas. Give it a shot because it works for me, and who knows how much benefit you could gain from using the same relaxation techniques.

EATING TO GET RID OF ECZEMA

As suggested earlier, there are lots of different foodstuffs and beverages to avoid, things that might cause your condition to flare up if you suffer from eczema.

On the other hand, if you want to reduce the more unpleasant effects of eczema, you should definitely include a variety of nutrients in your diet. To combat eczema, make sure your diet is high in the nutrients you require.

There are various different nutrient groups that are widely believed to offer great benefits to anyone who suffers from eczema.

The vitamin B complex: While it was once thought that there was only one type of vitamin B, it is now known that there are eight vitamins that together make up the vitamin B complex. While each form of vitamin B has its own health benefits, they also work together as a "team" to promote various aspects of essential health.

All of the individual components of the vitamin B complex cooperate with one another to help the body function in many different ways.

Of particular interest to an eczema sufferer is the fact that the vitamin B complex is known to boost metabolic function and to promote skin and muscle tone. Vitamin B also helps to support both the immune and nervous systems, while also promoting cellular rejuvenation, growth and division.

In short, including vitamin B complex in your diet will benefit your skin while also assisting your immune system in protecting your body so that it can fight skin conditions like eczema and psoriasis far more effectively. Bananas, lentils, potatoes, green vegetables, and Tempeh are all high in the various vitamins that comprise the vitamin B complex.

You can also find vitamin B in many other foodstuffs such as eggs and dairy products, but as we discovered earlier in this report, these may be foodstuffs that make your eczema problem worse, rather than better.

The alternative is to take vitamin B supplements to increase your daily intake of this essential vitamin. Whether this is a sensible or viable option will be determined in large part by whether eating enough 'natural' vitamin B. sources is a realistic option, because if not, supplementing your diet will be your best option.

Zinc: Zinc is a trace mineral that we all need in our diet because zinc possesses extremely powerful antioxidant qualities, which will help to prevent damage to or ageing of your skin.

Some foodstuffs that provide a reasonable level of zinc are things like lean roast beef, dates, roasted pumpkin and squash seeds.

The major problem with trying to consume enough zinc in your everyday diet is that most of the foods that are really rich in zinc are foods that you might be avoiding:

Zinc Rich Foods List	Milligrams	Portion
Oysters	25 +	100g
Shellfish	20	100g
Brewers Yeast	17	100g
Wheat Germ	17	100g
Wheat Bran	16	100g
All Bran cereal	6.8	100g
Pine Nuts	6.5	100g
Pecan Nuts	6.4	100g
Ok Sources of Zinc	Milligrams	Portion
Liver	6	100g
Cashew Nuts	5.7	100g
Parmesan Cheese	5.2	100g
Fish	3	100g
Eggs	2	100g

It may be necessary to find zinc supplements rather than trying to consume sufficient amounts of zinc in your normal daily food intake.

Fish oil: I mentioned earlier that fish oil is extremely important because of the widely accepted health benefits of omega-3 fatty acids. Fish oil, on the other hand, is a very rich source of vitamin A, which is necessary for maintaining healthy skin while also providing anti-inflammatory benefits. Given that eczema is a skin inflammation condition, including adequate amounts of vitamin A in your diet or supplemental nutrition program is critical.

Grape or cherry juice: Both of these juices possess antioxidant and anti-inflammatory qualities, so by doing nothing more complex than drinking a glass of juice every day, you could give your body a significant boost in its fight against eczema.

FIGHTING ECZEMA FROM THE INSIDE

There is evidence that eczema is caused by an immune system that is not as powerful or robust as it should be. As a result, using natural treatments and herbs to boost your immune system can help keep your eczema under control. There are numerous herbs that can improve the performance of your immune system, increasing your ability to fight eczema from the inside out. By incorporating or supplementing your diet with these herbs, you increase your chances of dealing with your eczema in a completely holistic manner.

Milk vetch

Milk vetch or Astragalus membranaceus is one of the most important plants in traditional Chinese medicine, one that has been used for at least 2000 years to strengthen the body.

When it comes to using Astragalus to treat eczema, the first thing to understand is that it is an adaptogen, which is a substance that helps the body de-stress both physically and psychologically. Knowing that stress can often play an extremely important part in causing eczema attacks, this ability to reduce stress naturally is extremely important.

Many studies of the effects of the milk vetch have indicated that the plant offers 'non-specific' immune system benefits. This means that instead of activating the body's defence system against one particular form of 'invader' or infection, it enhances the overall strength of the immune system by increasing the number of macrophages, the all-important white blood cells that give the immune system its strength and ability to resist attack.

Another significant advantage of Astragalus is that it has both tissue regenerating and anti-inflammatory properties. It provides a great deal of assistance to an eczema sufferer because it reduces inflammation and also helps healthy new skin tissue to grow.

With extremely powerful antibacterial qualities as well, Astragalus is definitely a herbal remedy that you must include in your diet.

In China, a piece of Astragalus root is boiled in a broth with ginseng and other health-giving plants before being discarded and served. This is not only highly nutritious, but also extremely tasty and an excellent way to incorporate milk vetch into your diet.

St John's wort

St. John's wort, also known as Hypericum perforatum, is a plant that contains a variety of compounds that have been shown to have numerous medical and psychological benefits. While St John's wort is best known for its ability to act as an antidepressant that is just as effective as pharmaceutical antidepressants like Prozac, it is also a herb that can help people with eczema. The ability to counteract depression and affect mood is extremely relevant. If this herb has the ability to counteract depression, it makes it far less likely that you will suffer the kind of stress related problems that can make your eczema problem flare-up at any time.

Going beyond this and without delving into every individual active constituent of St John's wort, its most obvious benefit for an eczema sufferer is that it is a very powerful anti-viral and antibacterial agent, which significantly boosts the strength of your immune system.

Because of these properties, it is also a highly effective herb for promoting rapid recovery from skin damage. For example, studies have shown that applying St John's wort topically to burns can help patients recover from their burn trauma up to three times faster than pharmaceutical applications.

Garlic

The active ingredient in garlic that gives it its distinctive pungent odor is allicin, a sulphur-rich volatile oil. This oil is responsible for garlic's ability to boost your immune system while also stimulating circulation and killing bacteria. In other words, garlic is another natural antibacterial substance that can help to improve the quality of your immune system, thereby strengthening your body's ability to reduce the severity and frequency of eczema flare-ups.

However, in addition to being extremely effective as an antibacterial agent, garlic has many other qualities that further boost your immune system to fight back against any kind of infections or medical conditions such as eczema or psoriasis. For example, garlic has been shown to be antiparasitic, anti-viral, antiseptic and antifungal.

In short, including a healthy dose of garlic in your diet is going to give your immune system a significant boost, which would in turn help your body to fight against eczema.

The only downside of eating lots of garlic every day is that some people might find your breath a little unpleasant, which could be inconvenient at those times when you want to be at your best.

As a result, many people who suffer from a variety of conditions, including eczema, prefer to take garlic capsules rather than eat garlic. There is nothing wrong with doing so, though it may influence your decision if you realize that including garlic in your diet is significantly less expensive than having to purchase a steady supply of garlic capsules. Nevertheless, no matter how include garlic in your daily 'diet', the main point is that you should do so as soon as possible.

Sage

Salvia officinalis is the full scientific name of the common sage that is most effective for treating skin conditions like eczema. The fact that we commonly refer to topical skin applications that are most soothing and reviving as'salves' should give you an idea of how effective this herb can be in assisting you with your eczema problem.

Sage is packed with powerful antioxidants, so it is highly effective in dealing with a condition like eczema. In addition, it has marked antibacterial qualities and is a known immune system stimulant.

According to available research, using sage as a component of herbal-based eczema potions for topical use as well as including it in your diet can reduce the severity of an eczema attack more quickly than almost any other herbal remedy, both applied to the skin and taken internally.

Honey

Honey is a natural antibacterial substance that is often classified as one of the 'super foods' because of its abilities to boost your immune system and increase your natural vitality and energy levels.

Although most people think of honey as a sweet substance produced by bees, you might be surprised to learn that honey is a complex mixture of antibacterial agents, organic acids, and a variety of trace minerals such as iron, copper, phosphorus, manganese, and zinc.

I previously highlighted that zinc is an essential element to include in your diet if you want to fight off eczema entirely naturally, so including honey in your daily food intake could be a very smart move indeed.

In fact, honey has many other properties that are especially beneficial to eczema patients. Surgical wound infections and skin burns, for example, respond remarkably well to topical applications of pure honey. Indeed, there is some evidence that burns respond better or faster to honey than to pharmaceutical burn treatments.

Not only should you include honey in your diet, but it is also something that you can apply topically to eczema affected areas of the skin to bring instant relief and to help reduce the chances of scarring.

Shitake mushrooms

Shitake mushrooms have been used in ancient Chinese medicine for thousands of years, and in modern Japan, they are used to help chemotherapy and radiation patients recover faster.

This is because the medicinal benefits of Shitake mushrooms have the ability to penetrate deep into the bone marrow of anyone who eats them on a regular basis.

An eczema sufferer will be more interested in the fact that one of the most important constituents of these mushrooms is lentinan. This substance has been shown to stimulate T-cell growth while also increasing macrophage activity, improving the strength and number of white blood cells, which are at the heart of a strong immune system.

Both of these characteristics are therefore highly relevant for boosting the performance of your immune system, as it is the ability of lentinan to increase production of immune competent cells.

Including Shitake mushrooms in your daily diet will therefore give your immune system a great deal more strength to fight back against eczema attacks in the future, so they are definitely something that should be added to your weekly shopping list.

OTHER HERBS FOR TREATING ECZEMA

Apart from the natural substances already mentioned in the chapter (all of which appear to provide significant benefits for eczema sufferers), many other herbal remedies have been reported by many sufferers to help alleviate the worst symptoms of eczema.

Most of these herbs should be applied to the eczema affected area of the skin, ideally after making a suitable oil compound with mild baby oil.

These herbs include burdock and licorice root, cleavers, nettles, yellow dock leaves and red clover.

Furthermore, lotions based on chamomile and/or primrose oil have provided relief to many sufferers, and we have previously considered both tea tree and olive oil for use as a topical treatment for eczema due to the antibacterial and soothing properties of both of these oils.

As suggested many times previously, there is no hard and fast rule about what will work for any individual eczema sufferer and what won't.

It is therefore a question of trying all of these solutions to see what works for you.

CONCLUSION

There are numerous natural approaches to treating eczema. While doctors will almost always recommend pharmaceuticals such as corticosteroids and antihistamines, there is no need to use potentially dangerous chemical drugs unless your eczema has progressed to the point where natural treatments are no longer effective.

Fortunately, for the vast majority of sufferers, this possibility is never likely to become a reality. The majority of people who suffer from eczema will have to put up with intense itching from time to time, but luckily, for most people, eczema is never likely to become dangerous.

As suggested, there is no way that even the most widely recognized eczema experts can claim that they fully understand the condition.

As the condition itself is not fully understood by the most eminent researchers and medical professionals themselves, it is almost impossible to state what will be effective in any particular case.

On the other hand, you have seen that there are numerous alternatives that you can try in your efforts to completely eliminate your eczema problem naturally.

As a result, if a natural solution does not appear to work, it is simply a matter of moving on to the next alternative natural treatment.

In this book, I have attempted to collect together as many natural eczema treatments as I could find, because I am aware that some treatments will work far better for some individuals than others.

The bottom line is that you now have plenty of natural treatments for eczema options available. There is no reason why you should delay before starting to try them.

www.ingramcontent.com/pod-product-compliance
Lightning Source LLC
Chambersburg PA
CBHW081833250726
48657CB00019B/3512